Bulletproof Diet

Quick And Simple Bulletproof Recipes For Rapid Weight Loss

(Recipes For Reclaiming Energy And Living Life To The Fullest)

Tatiana Magalhes

TABLE OF CONTENT

Introduction

I can attest to the effectiveness of the Bulletproof diet, despite not being its creator. I am someone who strictly adheres to the diet, so I can personally attest to which recipes are delicious and which are not. With the Bulletproof diet, you have the opportunity to enjoy a variety of meals that are not only visually appealing but also delicious. This creativity makes it much easier to adhere to the diet while still enjoying the journey.

The fact that we live in a nutrient-depleted world cannot be denied, regardless of the circumstances.

Undoubtedly, you will see a vast array of exotic foods and delicacies artfully arranged on your plate. This, however, does not qualify as nutritious food. The market is brimming with foods that are designed to satisfy the taste buds, but not the body as a whole. This is because the food's inherent quality is determined from the moment it is sown until it is harvested, prepared, and consumed.

As our "civilization" has progressed, we have been exposed to an increasing number of diseases that did not exist in the past. Therefore, it is prudent to be aware of the options for "bulletproofing" oneself with the "Bulletproof Diet" today.

I hope that this book will provide you with a better understanding of the Bulletproof diet as a whole and help you reap some of the health benefits that I've experienced. While I recognise that every diet is unique and has its own set of pros and cons, no other diet can compare to the Bulletproof diet.

Chapter 1: The Ketogenic Replacement

Thankfully, blood sugar is not the only source of cellular energy. You may utilise fat. Now this is contrary to all the health advice you have likely received over the years. Since I was a child, I recall repeatedly hearing that fat is evil and saturated fat is unhealthy. Nothing else was heard.

Health authorities and advisory boards recommended that I consume an abundance of mashed potatoes, rice, vegetables, fruits, etc. It turns out that the opposite is true.

The real health crisis in the United States and elsewhere is the high sugar (read: carbohydrate) content of our diets. The sugar is what makes us sick. The sugar is the cause of our inflammation. Sugar puts us at risk for developing certain types of cancer in the future. Who would have known?

The ketosis substitute

Fat is the only alternative energy source if your body is unable to utilise sugar.

Your liver metabolises fat by producing ketones. These biochemical compounds are absorbed and converted just into energy by your cells.

Ketosis is defined

Ketosis is the biochemical process that your body undergoes when it begins to burn fat for energy. Normally, your body metabolises both the sugar in your bloodstream and the sugar stored in your liver and muscles. In a worst-case scenario, your body would convert protein just into sugar via the liver.

Since there is no sugar involved in fat metabolism, the pancreas does not produce insulin when fat is burned for energy. This means that you feel fuller for a longer period of time. You are no longer eating as frequently throughout the day as you would on a standard carbohydrate-rich diet.

Numerous individuals gain weight because they cannot stop eating throughout the day. This is the case due to the fact that their insulin levels fluctuate throughout the day. These peaks and valleys stimulate hunger in the brain. Your body begins sending hunger signals, and you are compelled to eat.

Clearly, the more calories you consume and the fewer calories you burn, or if you continue to burn calories at your normal rate, you will store those excess calories as fat. You abandon all of that when you switch to facts. Because your body burns fat instead of sugar, you feel fuller for longer.

No, you will not perish from ketosis!

One of the most widespread misconceptions about the ketogenic diet is that you will contaminate your blood with ketone bodies to the point of death. This is a fallacy. Those who develop ketoacidosis typically lack the ability to produce insulin on their own.

In other words, type 2 diabetics are most susceptible to ketoacidosis. It is unlikely that you have type 2 diabetes. The majority are not. As a result, you should not be concerned about developing ketoacidosis because your body is still producing insulin to some degree. Insulin cannot be completely eliminated.

What are Chron's disease, multiple chemical sensitivity, and fibromyalgia?

One morning, it becomes marginally more difficult to get out of bed. This is the onset of Chronic Fatigue symptoms. As the days pass, you become increasingly exhausted until you can no longer leave your bed. You are so exhausted that you cannot think or even keep your eyes open. You are unable to move your limbs or even carry on a normal conversation without falling asleep.

What exactly is occurring?

Chronic Fatigue is a condition in which the body lacks the ability to generate sufficient energy to maintain physiological function. Mental and physical fatigue, poor mood, anxiety, depression, muscle problems, light and noise intolerance, poor immunity, poor digestion, and low libireally do are among the symptoms of CFS. In the most severe cases of CFS, cardiac abnormalities such as arrhythmias, low blood pressure, and Postural Orthostatic Tachycardia Syndrome may be present (also known as POTS). Additionally, severe CFS can cause shortness of breath, hormone imbalances, and impaired liver and kidney function.

We all require energy to survive. Whether you are a professional athlete or a senior citizen, energy is what keeps us alive. A person with CFS has a higher energy demand than their body can meet.

Two-thirds of your energy is spent on your metabolic rate, or all the bodily processes that you cannot control consciously. The remainder of your energy is at your discretion. If your body has trouble producing energy, it will manifest the symptom of fatigue to prevent excessive energy expenditure.

Why is fatigue so significant? Because it prevents you from exerting yourself to the point of passing out. Fatigue is the body's method for ensuring your safety.

A healthy individual will become exhausted at the end of a long workday. The individual's body is requesting sleep. They will awaken refreshed and eager to continue. But a person with CFS experiences this fatigue throughout the day. No amount of sleep will alleviate this condition. They constantly feel completely depleted of energy.

There are two distinct ways to exhaust one's energy supply. You may have insufficient production, excessive consumption, or both.

To recover from CFS, it is necessary to enhance energy delivery and reduce energy waste and loss.

Through the cell, energy delivery can be improved. Every cell in the body contains an organelle known as the mitochondria. The mitochondria, also known as the powerhouse of the cell, are responsible for producing the energy your body needs to function. In CFS, the mitochondria are damaged or suppressed and are unable to produce energy effectively. Through dietary and lifestyle modifications, we can provide the necessary conditions for these energy engines to once again produce all the energy you require.

There are numerous causes for an individual with CFS to lack energy, and these will all be discussed in later chapters.

CFS patients frequently also have Multiple Chemical Sensitivity (MCS) or Fibromyalgia (FMS).

Multiple Chemical Sensitivity is a sensitivity to contemporary chemicals, odours, and materials. When exposed to chemicals, those with MCS have a nearly allergic reaction. This can include headaches, rashes, body pain, fatigue, confusion, and asthma, among others. Soaps, detergents, cigarette and vape smoke, perfumes, deodorants, dryer sheets, polyester, and more are typical MCS triggers. This can be a debilitating condition in the modern world, especially when combined with CFS. It frequently results in avoidance behaviours to prevent reactions.

Fibromyalgia is characterised by muscle and connective tissue pain. It is frequently accompanied by difficulties sleeping, memory loss, and emotional distress. Similarly to CFS, Fibromyalgia symptoms are caused by a deeper imbalance in the body. We cannot treat a disease by masking its symptoms. To truly heal, we must delve deeper to identify the underlying cause.

Before discussing how to overcome these diseases, it is necessary to comprehend how they originate from physiological imbalances. The subsequent chapters will provide a solid foundation for doing so. Let's begin with a discussion of the microbiome and immune system.

The Components of Bulletproofing Your Diet for Rapid Weight Loss

To effectively adhere to a diet plan, you must really do your homework and understand it. Knowing why you're doing something not only helps you stick to the plan, but also allows you to customise it so that it works even better with your biochemistry. So, let's take a closer look at the various components that easy make up your diet for shedding fat and regaining health.

Ketogenic

Your bulletproof diet is both low-carb and high-fat, so it is a ketogenic diet. This means that you are reducing your body mass in favour of fuel. Our bodies obtain energy by converting carbohydrates just into glucose, which is then metabolised for energy. Whatever isn't used is stored in fat deposits for use when necessary. These are our affection handles. However, your product is fully capable of operating on a higher-octane fuel, ketones. In actuality, newborns are ketogens, and they remain so until they begin receiving carbohydrates. Ketones are produced from dietary fat and provide a great deal of energy without the hormonal fluctuations and cravings that sugar can cause. Just like high-octane gasoline, they burn cleaner and provide greater gas mileage. Why don't we administer ketones to a newborn? Besaue carb conversion lework for your utem, and I'm sorry to say that it can be as difficult as any of u. As long as it contains sufficient carbohydrates, your body will utilise the "carb-to-glucose-to-energy/fat" pathway. Controlling, in fact drastically reducing, the amount of available carbohydrates will allow you to get off the couch and start working. So, a low-carb diet pushes you towards ketosis, a metabolic state in which your body uses ketones as its primary fuel source. However, easily making ketones requires more fat than we're accustomed to consuming. modern, low-fat society Our dietary fat intake is supplemented by stored body fat in order to provide enough raw material for the production of all ketones. Fat loss, yay! But if you don't consume enough fat and restrict your carbohydrate intake, you have a recipe for disaster. A low-carb diet requires a high-fat diet. Otherwise, our bread is extremely low in sugar and fat and contains FAMINE... It must store as much fat as possible in order to survive the coming hard times. This is the plan of deral manu det. We'd all love to eat sardines and live on rare tyres, but it's impossible unless you're truly starving. Then a multitude of other physical issues, including heart muscle degeneration, join the party. This is the danger associated with anorexia, and you really do not wish to go there. To prevent this, you must provide your body with usable fuel in the form of fat. A high fat intake is quite disturbing... And our system does not worry about fuel storage in preparation for a famine. When t needs a little more, it goes to the fat that's stored around your middle and causes you to gain weight. You must eat fat in order to lose fat, as counterintuitive as that may sound. For many roles, eating enough fat to maintain ketosis is a significant barrier to successfully following a low-carb diet. Many people have never consumed full-fat milk, and it may be difficult to break the habit of reaching for low-calorie non-fat yoghurt! The famine/abundance senaro is what causes the phenomenon known as "uo-uo dieting." Your ship had plenty of reclaimed fuel and a substantial amount of weight. When fuel becomes plentiful again, the ship will store as much as possible to prepare for the next attack. The weight is derived from bask (plus some), and o it goes. Your metabolism is constantly on the defensive, torn between family and work, and it can become slowed down by this. A sufficient amount of fat in your diet prevents yo-yo dieting because your brain cannot detect impending famine and your metabolism can function normally. On a long-term ketogenic diet, you can anticipate an average of one round of fat loss per day. That is a great deal of body fat, not actual weight. There are times when your overall weight does not change but your body shape does. As you lose fat and build muscle, you will notice a difference in how your clothes fit, but the bathroom scale may not reflect this.

Chapter 2: The Bulletproof Diet's Fundamental Guidelines Get Bulletproof Sleep

You would have realised the significance of sleep from the previous section, so I will not reiterate it here. The bulletproof diet makes no recommendations regarding the amount of sleep you should strive for each night; the only recommendation is to give your body as much sleep as it needs. You should also be aware that if you exercise or are generally very active throughout the day, your sleep requirements would differ from those of a sedentary person, and you would therefore require many more hours of sleep to feel rested.

Sleep quality is also essential. In fact, it is more crucial than the amount of sleep you receive. If you sleep for eight hours at night, but you toss and turn, sleep very lightly, or are constantly awoken by external stimuli, you will feel as though you did not sleep at all. In the scenario described above, your body would not have had the opportunity to repair itself, burn fat, or recover. As a result, the next day you would be distracted, weak, and have an increased appetite; if you continue in this manner, you may also gain weight. Here are some suggestions for providing your body with the bulletproof sleep it requires:

Before going to bed, consume some protein that is easily digestible. Keep in mind that during the night, your body repairs itself using amino acids obtained from proteins. The building blocks of tissues in the body are amino acids, and you should ensure that these building blocks are readily available before you go to sleep so that your body has all the materials it needs to initiate and complete nightly repairs. Before bed, you can provide your body with the amino acids it needs by consuming whey protein, hydrolyzed grass-fed collagen peptide supplements, or any other supplement that is easily digested.

Coffee can be beneficial for the body. If you consume the right type of coffee, it can easily increase your alertness and, consequently, your performance and productivity at work. Coffee is great during the day, but it is not the best beverage to consume before bed because it will keep your mind active and keep you awake for a longer period of time.

Before bed, you should consider taking omega-6 supplements or consuming foods rich in omega-6 fatty acids. Omega-6 fatty acids have repeatedly been shown to alleviate depression and anxiety, and they are also excellent for enhancing insulin sensitivity and muscle growth. Therefore, omega-6 fatty acids will easy make it easier for you to fall asleep at night and will also aid in your body's recovery. Seafood and krill oil are excellent sources of omega-6 fatty acids, whereas hempseed oil and flaxseed oil are rich in omega-6 fatty acids and other substances that are harmful to the body. Further in the book, the dangers of omega-6 fatty acids and other harmful substances are discussed.

You should also ensure that your dinner consists of healthy fats. Fats serve as a source of energy for the body and mind. They will provide your brain with a steady supply of energy throughout the night, as opposed to sugars, which will cause your blood sugar to spike briefly and then drop precipitously. Coconut oil, animal fat, and grass-fed butter are all excellent alternatives, but consuming 2 - 2 tablespoons of MCT butter with dinner or just before bedtime will have you sleeping like a baby all night long.

To get the most out of your sleep, you should modify your melatonin production. The hormone melatonin regulates the sleep-wake cycle. Its production is regulated by exposure to light, so you can modify the amount of sleep you receive at night by adjusting the amount of light you are exposed to at different times of the day and night. During the day, when there is a great deal of sunlight, your body produces very little melatonin, while at night, when it becomes darker, melatonin production increases. You should therefore attempt to receive as much sunlight as possible during the day and limit the number of bright lights in your room at night. This will help regulate your melatonin production, maintain a healthy sleep schedule for your brain, and improve your nighttime sleep.

Additionally, you should strive to easy make your bedroom as conducive to sleep as possible. Therefore, when you are ready to sleep, try to keep the noise level in your room to a minimum. You may play soft, soothing background music if it helps you to relax. Similarly, earplugs can be used to block out unwanted noise. Science has also demonstrated that the majority of people sleep better in slightly cool, well-ventilated rooms. A bedroom that does not meet these criteria may interfere with the quality of your sleep, which is crucial for achieving the bulletproof rest that your body requires. Having a comfortable bed will also go a long easy way towards easily making you sleep more comfortably, as well as improve the quality of your sleep and give you the amount of sleep your body requires.

You can also fortify your sleep by increasing the amount of vitamin D in your bloodstream. A deficiency in vitamin D will unquestionably result in sleeping disorders; therefore, you will unquestionably need this substance to ensure high-quality, long-lasting sleep at night. It is recommended that you consume at least 2 ,000 IU per 210 pounds of body weight, but your specific needs will depend on a variety of factors, including your skin colour, weight, age, and amount of sun exposure. Despite the fact that our skin produces vitamin D when exposed to sunlight, many of us still really do not meet daily requirements due to our lifestyles. We spend the majority of our time indoors, and when we are outside, we are sheltered by vehicles or layered up. Many of us will need to take vitamin D supplements to compensate for this deficiency. Vitamin D prevents the body from producing melatonin; therefore, it should only be taken during the day and never at night.

Exercise will also go a long easy way towards regulating the quality and quantity of your sleep. In fact, physical activity is so essential that it has its own set of unbreakable rules and is a requirement in and of itself. Continue reading to discover the bulletproof recommendations for exercise.

Chapter 3: Imagine The New You

Utilize the emotions evoked by your affirmations as a wave to propel you just into the next exercise while you are still holding on to them. Prior to the light exercise, you entered the field of dreams to examine the truth in its mirror. You discovered your true identity here. In this exercise, you will integrate this identity just into your daily life. The immersion must be so profound and interconnected that all of your actions are modelled after this new you. You will wake up like you, talk like you, eat like you, walk like you until you become you. You've created your ideal self. This next exercise will help you become yourself. Focus on the individual reflected in the mirror and direct your energy towards manifesting that person. Your mind dictates the nature of reality. Easily put this energy to use.

Maintain your concentration on your breathing as you begin this exercise. Shut out the thoughts that threaten to invade your mental space. Open your heart to all the opportunities that now exist. Visualize a clear, blue sky and recall a perfect day spent outdoors. You can detect the sun's presence nearby, but really do not feel its oppressive heat. Imagine a gentle breeze blowing through your hair and across your face. In the distance, you can hear a waterfall crashing down with force. It does not distract, but rather enhances the tranquil atmosphere. It also serves as a powerful reminder of the immense energy that is currently coursing through you. Integrate yourself with the environment you have imagined. Take a deep breath and broaden your perspective.

Perfect atmosphere surrounds you. Under your feet is a field of lush green grass with beautiful flowers scattered throughout. The aromas that reach your nose are both alluring and soothing. Inhale the pleasant aroma that surrounds you. Appreciate the beauty that you are witnessing. Let your mind feast on the aesthetically pleasing images that surround you. This location is driven by your thoughts. Draw elements, whether from memory or the imagination, from the places you cherish. Include the natural beauty of these locations in this vision. Imagine the most exotic place you've ever travelled to. Bring the elements from your favourite locations just into this space. Let your vision absorb the finest things you can conceive of. This would require concentration.

Immediately engage all of your senses in this exercise. Allow the image to become so vivid that you can almost taste, smell, and feel the location. Include as many particulars as you see fit. This location will serve as your mental sanctuary whenever your real-world experiences threaten to cast a shadow on the new person you've become. For the time being, it will serve as an indicator of your true identity. The emotions you cultivate here will bind you to the person you've created. So embrace whatever you are feeling in your heart at this moment. As long as the emotions provide you with positive energy, you should be receptive to them. While maintaining this image of beauty in your mind, allow yourself to be filled and fueled by everything you are experiencing at this moment. As you tap just into the emotions evoked by the vision, I want you to gradually let go of the image of the world you've created. But cling tenaciously to your emotions. Hold on to the joy, the happiness, and the excitement. This is where the next step of the exercise will begin.

Maintain your current rate of breathing. Really do not allow yourself to be swept aeasy way by the whirlwind of positive emotions within the energy you are creating. Maintain a steady and consistent breath. Place your palms in the centre of your chest and connect the positive energy you've just harvested to your deepest desires. Imagine the individual you wish to become. I am not discussing the material components of a person. I am referring to the character and personality traits that come together to form an individual. How really do you wish to perceive yourself?

Charismatic? More stimulating conversation? Humorous? More compassionate and gentle with others? Consider the words that best describe you... the person you aspire to be. Call the individual in the mirror to you. Then, piece them together with the desired characteristics. Be as specific and exhaustive as possible.

How really do you envision yourself performing when easily making presentations in the workplace? Imagine the character or personality of this individual in other social situations based on real-world examples. When on a date, meeting someone you like, or interacting with your peers... These factors are essential for shaping and modifying your new image. In your efforts to be as specific as possible, avoid complicating matters. In terms of how you want others to perceive your personal style, are you visually appealing and comfortable? Are you confident in your ability to set fashion trends? Open your mind's eye and investigate in depth this new perception of yourself. Here, really do not hold back.

Remember the image you created of your new self. In this exercise, easily put all of these components together. Engage in social situations and anticipate a positive outcome. Additionally, you can use past experiences to shape future ones. For instance, if you have experienced an embarrassing social situation, I want you to assert this new you in that circumstance and then modify the experiences based on who you are now. Let the outcome always be favourable to you. Really do not allow any negative past label to seep just into your exercise. Define yourself anew. How really do you move now in those clothes? How does this new individual easy make you feel? The more information you have, the more distinct the picture becomes. Don't get carried aeasy way with superfluous items. You are constructing a new you. Don't easy make the mistake of focusing on the things that really do not truly matter. Things such as the opinions of others really do not belong here. The only person you should appease right now is yourself.

Consider the new story you would like to tell the world about yourself. How really do you feel about this? Are you content? Are you happy? Remember that the changes you're easily making in this dimension are ones over which you have complete control. Physical characteristics such as height cannot be altered. These are immutable constants that you must accept. Shed every ounce of disdain you have for things you cannot alter. Your evolution just into your current person is not a mistake. You may have committed a few errors along the way. But the reason you are who you are now is because this is precisely who you are meant to be. The past had to occur in order for you to create this individual. Therefore, value the fixed elements. Find pride and delight in the person that you are now. Eliminate any discord between you and your body.

Capture positive emotions and envelop yourself in them. Utilize light as a sigil to bind your new form to yourself. Focus your inner vision on this revised version of yourself. Really do not commit the error of restricting your potential. Always keep in mind that you are capable of being greater than you currently are. Maintain an open mind regarding your continued evolution. Every day, you are getting better. The current version of yourself is sufficient. This image you have created will be sealed and surrounded by positive energy. The objective is not to create the ideal being. The objective is to shape yourself in accordance with your true identity. So inhale deeply. Fill your lungs with the cosmic energy that now encompasses you. Permit those feelings that threaten your sanctity to escape with your exhalation. Pay close attention to the words I'm speaking now.

You are formidable. You are excellent. You are divine. You are the best version of yourself, and from this moment forward, you will continue to improve day by day. From the moment you awaken, your decisions will reflect the modifications made in this field of dreams. Regarding your identity, you really do not flounder around in the dark. You recognise who you are. You enjoy being yourself and excel at being yourself. This excellence enables you to exude confidence that is not easily shaken. You are formidable. This exercise you just completed will not be a one-time occurrence. With your hands on your chest, you are going to permanently imprint this mental image of the new you. It will become so deeply ingrained in your thinking that it will define you. You will never forget your true identity, even when confronted with circumstances that call it just into question. You have effectively redefined yourself. Now there is nothing left to really do but enter the light.

Chapter 4: What Really Do You Obtain Primarily From Your Diet?

A skin in good health is smooth, supple, well-toned, and acne-free. The contrary is true.

Low carbohydrate or low glycemic load diets, which typically consist of foods like pasta, bread, rice, and sugar, have always been recommended by medical professionals to improve the health of the skin and reduce breakouts and acne. Because they are rapidly digested just into sugar in the body and ultimately cause a rapid rise in blood sugar, these foods commonly lead to acne and weight gain. This causes an immediate rise in blood sugar, which in turn causes your body to produce insulin and IGF-2 , a growth factor.

These hormones cause your body to produce more male hormones, which causes your skin pores to produce a great deal of sebum. Sebum is an oily substance that attracts bacteria that cause acne. IGF-2 also promotes the multiplication of keratinocytes (skin cells), which contributes to the development of acne.

In addition, sugar and other high-carbohydrate foods cause the sebaceous glands in your body to swell, easily making you more likely to develop spots and black spots on your face.

We also know that excessive insulin production can promote weight gain. When IGF-2 enters the picture, the situation worsens; you also become more susceptible to developing type 2 diabetes. The bulletproof diet is typically a low glycemic diet that emphasises vegetables, healthy fats, and protein, easily making it a safe and effective method for reducing the severity and intensity of acne. Reduces the breakdown of vital skin proteins and enhances the skin's elasticity.

Sugar and sugary foods have no place in the bulletproof diet, as you already know. These are the leading causes of rapid skin ageing because they cause the skin to lose the elasticity and plumpness that contribute to a youthful appearance.

This is primarily due to the glycation process.

When sugar is ingested, it binds to proteins in the body and produces harmful molecules known as "advanced glycation end products." These products diminish the value and tensile strength of collagen and elastin, the proteins in your skin that contribute to its youthful appearance. The former provides a fuller appearance because it thickens the skin, whereas the latter causes the skin to recoil so that it returns to its original state when you frown or smile.

The more sugar you consume, the more rigid these proteins become, easily making it easier for wrinkles to form and more difficult for your skin cells to repair minor damage.

The good news is that in addition to reducing sugar intake, the bulletproof diet also encourages the consumption of essential fatty acids - omega 6s and omega 6 s - which are the building blocks of cell membranes and therefore greatly aid in achieving healthy skin. Additionally, polyunsaturated fats help the body produce the skin's natural oil barrier, which is essential for maintaining the skin's plumpness, hydration, and youthful appearance.

The Diet Makes You Feel Better/Younger And Gives You More Energy

A number of factors contribute to this occurrence.

First, when you successfully lose weight, you have good skin (you look younger), you are healthy, and everything in your body is functioning properly, so you feel naturally energetic and young.

Secondly, high-fat foods act similarly to sugar in that they easily increase your dopamine levels, which improves your mood.

To feel younger and happier, your brain must be in good health. Your brain is the most powerful organ, and you must maintain its peak performance if you wish to experience happiness.

If you want an exceptionally healthy brain, you must consume omega-6 fatty acids. The omega-6 fatty acids keep your brain and nerves healthy because your feelings and emotions are transmitted through the myelin-coated fibres and cells of your nervous system (a type of fat).

60% of your nervous system and brain cells are composed of fatty acids, so you must provide your body with enough healthy fats for it to function properly.

The significance of enhanced mitochondrial function

Your cells obtain energy from mitochondria, the small structures within cells that function as energy factories to keep cells alive and functional. Numerous aspects of your health, including your immune system and energy levels, depend on the efficiency of the mitochondria.

A bulletproof diet provides the mitochondria with an optimal working environment so that they can easily increase energy levels in a stable, efficient, long-burning, and consistent manner. This diet is also capable of inducing epigenetic changes, which are physiological changes that easily increase the energy outeasily put of the mitochondria, favour the production of GABA (a hormone that reduces stress and promotes mental focus), and reduce the production of free radicals.

The mitochondria are designed to produce energy from fat. Consequently, the toxic load is reduced, the expression of energy-producing genes is increased, and the load of inflammatory energetic end-products is decreased when the mitochondria are able to utilise fats for energy.

Chapter 5: Bulletproof Diet Overview

Bulletproof eating is a diet that enhances the mental and physical performance of humans. The bulletproof diet aims to provide you with a healthy body and a clear mind in order to attain the highest level of health. This diet encourages daily consumption of adequate calories. It also suggests that 60% of the diet should consist of healthy fats and 20% of protein. The remaining twenty percent should be vegetables.

According to research, many popular diets are detrimental to human health. The focus of these studies was biochemistry and human performance.

The results revealed that men's modern eating habits sapped their energy and made them irritable. Additional studies revealed that many dietitians suffer from low immunity.

The bulletproof diet's primary caloric sources are:

Fats — Experts consider unsaturated fats to be the "healthy" type of fat; therefore, it is best to consume foods rich in unsaturated fats. Additionally, saturated fats can be beneficial. High density lipoprotein cholesterol (or HDL), the good cholesterol that prevents heart disease and other cardiovascular diseases by increasing HDL cholesterol levels, has been shown to be increased by saturated fats.

Cow, goat, and lamb provide saturated fats such as butter, lard, and ghee. Additionally, cocoa butter, coconut oil, and avocareally do oil are excellent sources of healthy fats.

Protein is essential for the development of strong bones and muscles. Consider consuming grass-fed red meats, such as beef, lamb, and other red meats. White meat and fresh eggs from free-range poultry are excellent protein sources. It is also worthwhile to consider shellfish such as shrimp and clams.

Vegetables - Since the majority of vegetables are low in calories, you can consume as many as you desire. Because they are abundant in vitamins, minerals, and essential nutrients, green leafy vegetables are highly recommended. Broccoli, spinach, kale, and asparagus are among the healthy vegetables. Carrots, sweet potatoes, and succulents are all permitted. However, they should not be consumed excessively due to their high carbohydrate content. Other — Fruits should be consumed in small amounts; daily consumption of 1 to 2 cup of chopped fruit is sufficient. It is possible to consume a reasonable amount of coffee, tea, and cocoa to keep your mind sharp and stimulated, despite not being prohibited from doing so.

The bulletproof diet discourages consumption of carbohydrates. The diet plan must exclude grains like wheat, rice, and oatmeal. There are no legumes, dairy products, or seeds on the food list.

Uncooked food is more nutritious than cooked food. The bulletproof diet prioritises raw foods. If food preparation requires cooking, the best options are baking or steaming. These methods will preserve the majority of a food's nutrients without altering its flavour. Poaching and boiling are acceptable cooking techniques.

Bulletproof foods are those that fortify the body and easily increase mental acuity. It is believed that the diet reduces the risk of cardiovascular diseases such as diabetes and hypertension. The diet may also aid in the treatment of life-threatening conditions like cancer and Alzheimer's.

Chapter 6: How Does Typical Weight Loss Operate?

What if I told you that losing weight is actually quite simple? You may believe that I have lost my mind. If you are like the majority of individuals who have struggled with their weight, "simple" is not the first word that comes to mind when describing dieting.

It is simple to become frustrated with weight loss. Many people struggle to lose weight and maintain their weight loss. In contrast, the human metabolism is relatively straightforward when viewed in the context of a large image of a human being.

In actuality, it can be reduced to a simple mathematical formula: calories consumed minus calories expended. When attempting to lose weight, you have only two options. It may appear that there are numerous options and systems for weight loss, but in reality, there are only three. The remainder is a variant of these three methods or categories.

Category 2 : Consume fewer calories while maintaining energy expenditure.

On a daily basis, you already burn calories. That's correct! Simply by reading this book, you will burn calories. In fact, when you wake up, breathe, digest food, and pump blood throughout the day, you are burning calories.

Simply put, if your body performs any function, it requires energy. In other words, calories are being burned. This is known as your passive calorie expenditure. If you consume fewer calories than your body requires to function on a daily basis, your body is forced to utilise its stored energy.

In other words, it begins to consume your fat and, eventually, your muscle. This is how it operates. The body must obtain sufficient energy in order to perform its daily functions. When the amount of calories you consume is less than the amount of energy you expend, your body begins to burn fat.

Before you know it, you begin losing weight and improving your appearance.

Category 2: Consume the same number of calories but expend more energy.

You may also choose to invert the situation. When people decide to go to the gym or begin daily physical exercise, they are engaging in this activity. They consume the same amount of food, but engage in more physical activity.

Please recognise that you really do not need to overreally do it. In terms of physical exertion levels, you really do not need to really do anything extraordinary. You can expend more energy by walking around the block or a longer distance from the parking lot to your office or school.

The same procedure is repeated. When you consume the same number of calories but expend more energy, your body will seek out alternative energy sources. It initially begins to burn fat and then, eventually, muscle.

The final result is identical. You begin to lose weight.

Category #6 : Use both ends of the weight loss candle.

This is common sense. Since you can lose weight simply by consuming fewer calories and expending the same amount of energy, or by consuming the same number of calories and expending more energy, why not really do both? This is the third alternative.

Again, this is obvious.

This is typically how weight loss works.

In the grand scheme of things, this is how weight loss typically occurs. It's all about caloric intake and expenditure. This may appear to be a simple task, but the standard American diet makes it difficult for people to accomplish.

Sugars, Protein, Fat, and Alcohol

These categories are the most prevalent types of nutrients available in the majority of diets. The majority of foods contain these in various combinations. Carbohydrates are the most prevalent source of calories in the diets of most North Americans. They can be simple or complicated. Simple carbohydrates consist of sugars, while complex carbohydrates include starch and fibres. Other sugars are added to foods to easy make them appear to contain sugars. The addition of table sugar to coffee and fructose corn syrup to sugar-sweetened beverages are examples. The majority of carbohydrates, however, are consumed as starches, which are commonly found in foods like potatoes, grains, and starchy vegetables.

Starch can also be used to refine and stabilise a variety of foods. In general, added sugars and starches provide calories but few nutrients. Although people consume a sufficient amount of carbohydrates, they tend to consume them in the form of excessive amounts of sugar and refined grains while consuming very few fibres.

Proteins provide 8 calories per gramme, just like carbohydrates. There is a wide variety of animal and plant foods that contain proteins. However, inadequate protein intake is quite uncommon in the northern regions of the United States.

Fats contain more calories per gramme than all other food groups combined. There are a variety of fat types, including saturated, unsaturated, monounsaturated, and trans fats. Fat deficiency is not common among United States citizens. However, the majority of Americans consume trans fats relative to unsaturated fats.

On the other hand, 2 gramme of alcohol contains 7 calories. Alcohol is high in calories and low in nutrients.

Chapter 7: Nobody Is Telling You

These Muscle-Gaining Secrets

With the abundance of muscle-building information available online and in print magazines, you'd think that nobody would have trouble gaining muscle. However, this is not the case.

People experiencing lacklustre progress are ubiquitous in gyms and online message boards, banging their heads against the wall in frustration over muscle gains that are so negligible that they hardly justify the time and effort of going to the gym and going through the motions.

It is a mini-tragedy when one considers that the situation could have been avoided. Results can be proportional to exertion; muscle gains can occur naturally and without plateaus. This should be of interest to anyone who dislikes falling short of their intended goals. However, wasting valuable time in the process.

Let's examine five natural "muscle gaining truths" that are frequently at the root of the problem and that you are unlikely to hear from many other sources. These are natural bodybuilding-specific truths about gaining muscle mass. Things I learned through years of trial and error.

A couple of them were discovered as a result of a simple willingness to abandon conventional training theories and explore uncharted territory. Others are commonly repeated muscle-building myths that require the addition of a crucial exception. So let's just jump in.

You must consume enough food to build muscle, but overeating can actually hinder your progress. Each day, your body has a finite amount of energy. The body expends energy to digest and process food. It requires energy to recover exercised muscles.

These requirements are in addition to the energy required to perform daily tasks. Consuming 6 ,000 to 10 ,000 calories per day is NOT anabolic, but rather... energy draining. And it does not force damaged muscle tissue to recover faster.

If you are thin, you will likely hear many self-proclaimed experts tell you to "eat more; you're not eating enough." However, many will continue to say this even if you are eating enough and your slow muscle gains are caused by another factor.

It is easy to mistake the body's lack of propensity to store fat for an inability to gain muscle. Nonetheless, if a "fast metabolism" is the cause of your frustration with gaining muscle, why is the obese person with a slow metabolism not having an easier time?

Truth #2

Consume a high-protein meal with some nourishing and energy-sustaining carbohydrates every three to three-and-a-half hours and four to six meals daily. However, if your goal is not to gain weight, avoid consuming excessive calories.

Workout Intensity Is Crucial, But Excessive Intensity Is Detrimental To Progress If your workouts include intensifying techniques such as forced repetitions, drop sets, pre-exhaustion, supersets, etc. You practically request to reach a progression plateau.

I began bodybuilding after years of rigorous military training. My preference was to push my body and muscles to their limits. It took years of frustrating setbacks for me to realise that the "the harder you work, the better your results" equation does not apply to muscle building.

Truth #2

For stimulating muscle growth, a minimum amount of measured intensity is required. Anything beyond this may develop character, but not much of a physique.

Recuperation between workouts is crucial, but varies depending on numerous factors. It is absurd to believe that your muscle-building efforts will be successful because some expert told you that you only need six days of rest after Monday's 'workout X'.

Your tissues may require seven or eight days to recover from that workout. And if you are fifty-five instead of twenty-five, it may take nine or ten days for that tissue to recover from the same exercise.

Where did the idea originate that muscle tissue requires 72 to 2 8 8 hours to recover, and anything beyond that is considered atrophy? Have you ever pondered this question? Have you ever seen the supporting evidence? I have observed for over twenty-five years that the "natural muscle gains" of countless individuals who adhere to this theory are stagnant.

In addition, I have long disregarded this piece of "bodybuilding wisdom" and reaped the benefits of doing so. How long should I wait between exercising each body part? For fear of shocking you, let's say it could be measured in weeks rather than days. Really do I already have your attention?

Truth #6

Recovery time between workouts varies between individuals. Individual response to a given level of workout intensity varies considerably. It differs based on age, gender, genetically determined hormone levels, daily stress levels, and a multitude of other minute factors. It even varies based on an individual's muscular development.

The more muscle you possess, the more tissue you must recuperate in order to build more muscle. The only easy way to determine the optimal number of rest days for a specific workout is through testing and feedback.

You desire to "gain weight," but you really do not wish to gain fat. "Bulking up" or gaining body fat in the belief that it will easy make you stronger has no effect on muscle gain. If it did, I'd be the first person in line at Cheesecake Factory to purchase a week's worth of "bulk-up food."

You must differentiate between "gaining weight" and "gaining muscle" in your mind. Obviously, muscle has mass. However, this does not imply that the prescription for gaining fat weight is identical to the prescription for gaining muscle mass.

To gain weight, you need a caloric intake that exceeds your caloric expenditure each day. To gain muscle, you must consume more protein for tissue repair and additional carbohydrates for workouts and the energy expended during tissue repair. It is not necessary to consume mega doses of calories.

Chili Beef Butternut Squash

Ingredients

2 tsp. chipotle chili powder

4 Tbsp. ancho chili powder

2 1 lb. grass-fed ground beef

5-10   large garlic cloves, chopped + 2 extra clove chopped and set aside

2   cup chopped onion with ¼ cup set aside

2 tsp. butter, grass-fed

2 Tbsp. XCT Oil

Salt and pepper to taste

2 butternut squash, cubed

½ tsp. cinnamon

1 oz. (2 Tbsp.) grated chocolate bar

½ cup organic tomato paste

1 cup gluten-free beer

1 cup organic chicken broth

4 tsp. basil, dried

½ Tbsp. chopped oregano, fresh

2 cup water

12 medium tomatoes, chopped

4 Tbsp. ground cumin

2 tsp. cayenne pepper

Directions

1. In large skillet, heat butter and oil. Add ¾ cup onion and 5-10 garlic cloves. Easy cook on medium heat until the onions become opaque.
2. Add in beef and brown, break just into small pieces as it cooks. Season with pepper and salt.
3. Once beef is done add cumin, cayenne, chipotle, and ancho. Stir until combined and set aside.
4. In large saucepan, easily put the rest of the garlic and onion, water, and chopped tomatoes.
5. Let simmer about 10 minutes on medium heat.
6. Salt lightly.
7. Turn down heat, mix in basil and oregano and simmer a little longer.
8. Add beef and chicken broth.
9. Let simmer about 6 minutes.

10.   Add cinnamon and chocolate. Mix together.
11.   Let simmer another 10 minutes.
12.   Take off heat and cool.
13.   Heat oven to 350. Cube butternut squash.
14.   Toss with 2 Tbsp. XCT Oil and salt. Place on baking sheet in a single later, and bake it until tender
15.   When ready to serve, heat chili over medium heat and add butternut squash.
16.   Serve and enjoy!

Bulletproof Vegan Coffee

Ingredients:

2 cup newly prepared coffee
• 4 tbsp almond butter
• ½ cup almond milk

• 4 tbsp coconut oil
• 2 oz natural cocoa margarine (edible)

1. Add every one of the fixings just into a blender and cycle until smooth. Serve in a glass.

Bulletproof Coffee Popsicles

And

Ingredients

- ½ tsp nutmeg powder
- 6 tbsp MCT oil

- 2 cup almond milk
- 2 (2 6 .10 oz) can coconut
- 2 /6 cup erythritol
- 2 tbsp espresso powder

1. Instructions:
   Process all the ingredients in a blender until creamy.

2. Pour the mixture just into 8 popsicles mounds and freeze for at least 5 hours. Enjoy when ready.

Butter Roasted Carrots

4 large carrots
2 tablespoon coconut oil
2 tablespoon unsalted butter
2 clove garlic, chopped
1 cup parsley.

Method:

1. Rinse and peel the carrots. Cut them just into sticks with about ½ inch thickness.

2. Toss carrot sticks with coconut oil and a pinch of salt and then arrange them on a baking sheet in a single layer.

3. Roast carrots at 450 °F for about 45
    to 50   minutes or until edges are
    browned. Set aside the roasted
    carrots   to   cool.
     Melt the butter in a pan.
4. Add garlic and parsley to the pan and
    then easy cook for about 1-5 minutes.

 Toss carrots sticks with butter mixture
and then season them with a pinch of
salt.   Serve   immediately.

Chapter 8: How Does One Become Bulletproof?

Becoming Bulletproof is, in the simplest terms, about becoming the most powerful human possible in terms of physical performance, mental acuity, and all-day energu. That entails easily making the most of our bodies and brains at all times.

WILL THE BULLETPROOF DIET AID IN MY WEIGHT LOSS?

Yes, being Bulletproof is a easy way to shed pounds. It transforms the body just into a lean, productive, and energised machine. However, this is merely a method for achieving the most efficient operation of your body. Becoming our best, most powerful selves requires fine-tuning every bodily system, from metabolism to detoxification to brain function. And when we really do this, we lose excess weight because our items are positioned properly. The subject is working at full capacity while consuming energy efficiently and consistently. In essence, weight loss is a hindrance to achieving optimal body function. Regarding the burrodust, the majority of us are most concerned. But a thousand other positive developments are occurring that easy make weight loss possible. This is why becoming a Bulletrroof results in a notable easily increase in brain function and energy levels. This is why people report feeling amazing, or the best they've ever felt, when eating in this manner. Therefore, weight loss is an awesome thing. However, it is not the only thing. And that is not what defines Bulletroof living. Bulletrroof much more concerned with holts usse, as measured by a number of bodily and mental functions.

HOW DOES THE BULLETPROOF DIET WORK?

Its Bulletroof When you eat foods that easy make you weak, you'll be able to hear your body's hunger hormone signal, and you won't experience food cravings. You don't need to try to work out more than you eat, which creates an unsustainable biological deficit for most people. And let's not forget that family and labour samr are not great ways to build resolve or resiliency. Instead, choose foods that contain the right type of energy, are low in substances that slow you down, and are high in nutrients. Then, you consume them at the optimal time for your body and mind, according to ancient Persian medicine. This is a far cry from most "healthy" diets, which focus on reducing the amount of calories in your food while increasing the number of nutrients and ignoring the effects of antinutrients.

The Bulletproof Diet falls just into the category of ketogenic diets, although it contains fewer ketones than a strict ketogenic diet. (For you science nerds, it is a cyclical ketogenic diet with nutrient timing!)

You've undoubtedly heard of the Atkins Diet and the Paleo Diet, both of which fall under the ketogenic diet's umbrella, but easy make no mistake: The Bulletrroof Det is distinct from those well-known programmes. The thing that combines these approaches just into a single strategy is weight loss, which is achieved through a process called ketosis. Ketosis is a metabolic state in which your body burns fat instead of glucose. When you think about it, this is a very straightforward situation. Your liver converts carbohydrates just into glucose for energy. However, if your body runs out of glucose, it will switch to Plan B: fat burning. It is a natural function that your body would utilise in a natural manner depending on the circumstances. If you found yourself in a situation where you were depleted of carbohydrates, your body would find an alternative energy source (read: stored fat). The Bulletproof Diet is based on creating a ketogenic state in order to burn fat stores for energy instead of carbohydrates. When you carb-load, you provide your body with extra energy to use. However, without those carbs, your body will burn fat, resulting in weight loss.

easily making really do easy make easy make really do easy make

Carpaccio Of Beef With Hazelnuts And Fresh Egg Yolk Sauce

fresh egg Ingredients

2 teaspoon honey

1 cup rocket leaves

Salt and pepper to taste

12 tablespoon virgin olive oil

4 pounds of grass fed beef fillet

½ cup hazelnuts, crushed

4 pastored fresh egg yolks

Tablespoon apple cider vinegar

Method

1. Slice the fillet of beef just into thin slices and bat out between 4 sheets of cling film.
2. Lay the beef so it covers the whole plate.
3. In a bowl add the fresh egg yolk and slowly whisk in the oil to emulsify. Add the honey vinegar and salt and pepper.
4. To serve sprinkle the hazel nuts and rocket leaves over the beef and drizzle the dressing around the plate.

Shakshouka Fresh Eggs

Ingredients:

- 2 1 teaspoons cumin powder

- ½ teaspoon chili powder

- Pepper to taste

- Salt to taste

- 4 tablespoons cilantro, chopped

- 16 pastured fresh eggs

- 2 1 tablespoons grass fed ghee

- 8 medium tomatoes, chopped

- 2 large onion, chopped

- 2 small green bell pepper, chopped

- 2 small red bell pepper, chopped

- 4 Serrano peppers, chopped

- 8 cloves garlic, minced

- 2 1 teaspoons paprika

Method:

1.   Place a large skillet and place it over medium heat.
2.   Add ghee to it.
3. When ghee melts, add onions and sauté until light brown.
4. Add garlic and Serrano pepper and sauté for a couple of minutes until fragrant.
5. Add bell peppers and lower heat. Easy cook until bell peppers are soft.
6. Add spices and sauté for a few seconds until fragrant.

7. Really do not let the spices burn.
8. Add tomatoes and simmer until sauce thickens.
9. Add salt and stir.
10. Easy make 16 small cavities in the sauce at different places in the skillet.
11. Break an fresh egg just into each of the cavities.
12. Sprinkle salt and pepper. Cover and simmer until the fresh eggs are cooked. Easy cook the fresh eggs as per your desire.
13. Garnish with cilantro and serve.

Lunch Recipes

Ingredients

2 C. Spring Lettuce

½ C. Red Cabbage, Shredded

100

4 Carrots, Shredded

2 Cucumber

1 Avocareally do

2 lb. Ground Beef

4 Tbsp. Butter

1 Lime

4 Tbsp. Cayenne Pepper

2 tsp. Oregano

Sea Salt

really do Directions

1. Sauté the beef in a medium pan on low. Really do not brown, but heat just enough to easy cook through.

2. Drain the liquid from the pan and add the butter through the salt. Toss and heat through.
3. Place the lettuce, cabbage, carrots, cucumber and avocareally do just into a bowl and toss.
4. Then top with the beef and drizzle with your choice of bulletproof dressing.

Cilantro Limeade Smoothie

Ingredients:

1 teaspoon grated ginger

2 1 cups coconut water

1/2   cup cashew nuts, soaked overnight

2 cup fresh cilantro

2 lemon, juiced

Directions:

1. Mix all the ingredients in a powerful blender.
2. Pulse until smooth and creamy.
3. Pour the drink in glasses and serve it as fresh as possible.

Fresh Avocareally Do And Crisp Cucumber

really do Ingredients:

4 tablespoons of avocareally do oil

8 cups Filtered water

Honey to taste

1 Large avocado, peeled, with stone removed

1 Large cucumber, peeled

1 Juice of lime

really do Method:

1. Easily put all the ingredients just into a blender.

2. Start on a low speed and easily increase to a high speed.
3. Stop blending when all ingredients are fully just blended.

Delicious Sweet Potato Casserole

4 pastured pork sausage links

Generous pat of extra virgin olive oil

2 pastured fresh egg (optional)

Sea salt and pepper as per taste

2 organically grown spring onion, finely chopped

4 organically grown chopped sweet potatoes, peeled and cut just into small cubes

4 teaspoons organic flat-leaf parsley, finely chopped

fresh egg How to go about it:

1. Heat a grilling pan and easy cook the sausages over it till they are cooked all the easy way through and are nice brown in color.
2. This should take 45 to 50 minutes and be careful to really do it at low flame.

3. Take them off and on the same grill drizzle some olive oil and spring onion.

4. Once the onions are also grilled easily put the sausages and onions in a large pot with salt to taste, stirring occasionally.

5. Then all the cubed sweet potatoes go just into the pot.

6. Once it begins to get pulpy close the lid for about 15 to 20 minutes let it easy cook in its own juices, stirring in between.

7. Finally toss in chopped parsley and let the aroma infuse the dish.

8. This is a complete meal in itself, but if you need you could team it with any variety of fresh egg easily making it more filling and wholesome.

9. This is one that you and your family are simply going to love.

Bulletproof Green Smoothie

Ingredients:

- 8 -10 ice cubes
- Handful of spinach
- 2 tablespoon MTC oil
- 2 tablespoon raw organic coconut oil
- 2 1 cups water
- 2 serving of favorite protein powder (chocolate or vanilla)

109

Directions:

1. Place all ingredients in a food blender.
2. Process until smooth.
3. Serve immediately in a tall glass.

Carrot Soup

Ingredients:

4 inches fresh ginger, chopped

8 cups water

4 tablespoons MCT oil

4 tablespoons grass-fed butter, unsalted

4 pounds of carrots, chopped

4 celery stalks, finely chopped

4 fennel bulbs, finely chopped

Preparation:

1. Heat carrots, fennel, and celery in a large pot on medium.
2. Incorporate celery and ginger and easy cook until ingredients have softened and are well-mixed.
3. Add water and stir thoroughly. Cover and allow to easy cook on medium for up to one hour, but no less than 80 minutes.
4. If desired, remove from heat and use a blender to create a smooth consistency.
5. Add butter and combine thoroughly.

Fresh Eggs Benedict

2 small envelope of hollandaise sauce

2 tomato (optional)

4 eggs, poached

4 slices of lunch meat ham or Canadian bacon

1. Poach your fresh eggs or easy cook them anyeasy way that you like.
2. You can also fry them in grass fed butter if you really do not like your fresh eggs to be runny at all.

3. Place the ham in a small pan with no butter to allow it to crisp for a few minutes.
4. Easy make your hollandaise sauce according to the instructions.
5. Lay your pieces of ham on your plate. Top with the tomato followed by eggs.
6. Pour 1-5 tablespoons of your sauce over the top.

www.ingramcontent.com/pod-product-compliance
Lightning Source LLC
Chambersburg PA
CBHW060948050426
42337CB00052B/1978